Contents

1.3 Understanding Weight Loss

Weight loss is a topic that has captivated the attention of millions of people around the world. While many individuals desire to lose weight, there is often confusion and frustration surrounding the process. This book aims to demystify weight loss by providing you with a clear understanding of its underlying principles.

In the first section of the book, "The Science of Weight Loss," we will delve into the intricate mechanisms that govern our body's ability to store and burn fat. We will explore the concept of caloric balance and how energy intake relates to energy expenditure. Additionally, we will discuss the role of metabolism and various hormones in regulating weight and uncover the factors that can influence these processes.

Setting Realistic Goals

One of the keys to successful weight loss is setting realistic and achievable goals. In this book, we emphasize the importance of goal setting and guide you through the process of establishing targets that are both motivating and attainable. We will help you determine your starting point and assess your current state by evaluating metrics such as body mass index (BMI), body composition, and waist circumference.

By setting realistic goals, you can maintain a positive mindset and track your progress effectively. We will provide you with strategies to establish short-term and long-term goals that align with your individual needs and preferences. Remember, weight loss is a personal journey, and the goals you set should be tailored to your unique circumstances and aspirations.

Throughout this book, we aim to equip you with the knowledge, tools, and support necessary to embark on a successful weight loss journey. We encourage you to approach this process with patience, determination, and a growth mindset. With the right mindset and a solid foundation of understanding, you can achieve sustainable weight loss and transform your life for the better.

In the subsequent sections of this book, we will explore various topics such as building a healthy eating foundation, identifying the best foods for weight loss, overcoming obstacles and challenges, and maintaining weight loss in the long term. Each section will provide valuable insights, practical tips, and actionable steps to support your weight loss goals.

Remember, you are not alone on this journey. By reading this book, you have taken an important step towards making positive changes in your life. So, let's embark on this transformative adventure together and embrace the incredible possibilities that lie ahead. Are you ready? Let's begin!

Creating a Personalized Weight Loss Plan

4.1 Identifying Your Motivation and Commitment

Embarking on a weight loss journey requires a strong sense of motivation and commitment. Before diving into specific strategies and techniques, it is crucial to identify the underlying reasons why you want to lose weight and the level of dedication you are willing to invest in achieving your goals.

Motivation serves as the driving force behind your weight loss journey. It can stem from a desire to improve your health, enhance your self-confidence, or simply feel better in your own skin. Take some time to reflect on your personal motivations for weight loss. Write them down and keep them in a place where you can revisit them whenever you need a reminder of why you started this journey.

In addition to motivation, commitment is equally important. It involves making a conscious decision to prioritize your weight loss goals and make the necessary lifestyle changes. Recognize that this journey will require effort, discipline, and perseverance. Commitment means staying dedicated even when faced with challenges or setbacks.

By understanding your motivation and solidifying your commitment, you lay the foundation for long-term success. Keep your motivation at the forefront of your mind as you move forward and use it as a source of inspiration during challenging times.

4.2 Setting Realistic and Achievable Goals

Setting realistic and achievable goals is crucial for sustaining motivation and making meaningful progress. While it's natural to have ambitious weight loss aspirations, it's important to set goals that are attainable within a reasonable timeframe. Unrealistic goals can lead to disappointment and frustration, undermining your motivation and potentially derailing your progress.

To set effective goals, follow these guidelines:

Be specific: Define your goals clearly. For example, instead of saying "I want to lose weight," specify the amount of weight you want to lose and the timeframe in which you aim to achieve it.

Make them measurable: Ensure your goals are quantifiable so that you can track your progress. For instance, set a goal to lose a specific number of pounds or inches.

Set a timeframe: Establish a realistic timeframe for achieving your goals. This will help you stay focused and motivated. Remember that healthy weight loss occurs at a rate of 1-2 pounds per week.

Break them down: Divide your long-term goals into smaller, short-term milestones. Celebrating these smaller victories along the way will keep you motivated and engaged.

Consider non-scale victories: Weight loss is not solely about the numbers on the scale. Set goals related to non-scale victories such as increased energy levels, improved sleep, or fitting into a certain clothing size.

By setting realistic and achievable goals, you create a roadmap for success. Regularly reassess and adjust your goals as you progress to ensure they remain challenging yet attainable.

4.3 Choosing the Right Diet Approach

When it comes to weight loss, there is no one-size-fits-all approach. Different dietary strategies work for different individuals. It's important to find a diet approach that aligns with your preferences, lifestyle, and health considerations.

Consider the following factors when choosing the right diet approach for you:

Nutritional balance: Opt for a diet that provides a balance of macronutrients (carbohydrates, proteins, and fats) and incorporates a variety of whole, unprocessed foods. Avoid extreme or restrictive diets that eliminate entire food groups.

Sustainable habits: Look for a diet approach that you can maintain in the long term. It should promote sustainable habits and be adaptable to different situations and social settings.

Individual preferences: Consider your food preferences, cultural background, and any dietary restrictions or allergies. Choose a diet that allows for flexibility and enjoyment of food while still supporting weight loss.

Professional guidance: Consult with a registered dietitian or nutritionist who can provide personalized recommendations based on your unique needs and goals.

Remember, the most effective diet approach is one that you can adhere to consistently and enjoyably over time. Be open to experimentation and be willing to modify your approach as needed.

4.4 Incorporating Physical Activity and Exercise

While diet plays a significant role in weight loss, physical activity and exercise are essential for overall health, improved fitness, and increased calorie expenditure. Incorporating regular exercise into your weight loss plan can enhance your results and contribute to long-term weight maintenance.

When choosing an exercise routine, consider the following:

Types of exercise: Include a combination of cardiovascular exercises (e.g., walking, running, cycling) and strength training (e.g., weightlifting, bodyweight exercises). This combination helps burn calories, build lean muscle mass, and improve overall fitness.

Personal preferences: Select activities that you enjoy and find motivating. Whether it's dancing, swimming, hiking, or playing a sport, engaging in activities you like increases the likelihood of sticking with your exercise routine.

Frequency and duration: Aim for at least 150 minutes of moderate-intensity aerobic exercise or 75 minutes of vigorous-intensity aerobic exercise per week. Additionally, incorporate strength training exercises two to three times a week to build and maintain muscle mass.

Gradual progression: Start at a comfortable level and gradually increase the intensity, duration, or frequency of your workouts. This gradual progression allows your body to adapt and helps prevent injury.

Lifestyle integration: Look for opportunities to incorporate physical activity into your daily routine. Take the stairs instead of the elevator, walk or bike to work if possible, or engage in active hobbies during your leisure

time.

The Biggest Loser Diet: Does It Work for Weight Loss?

The Biggest Loser diet is an at-home weight loss program inspired by the reality television show of the same name.

The plan claims to transform your body via healthier eating and exercise habits, including a strict low calorie regimen.

Still, you may wonder how effective it is.

This article tells you whether the Biggest Loser diet is a good choice for weight loss.

BOTTOM LINE: The Biggest Loser eating plan promotes weight loss by restricting calories and encouraging a diet comprising nutrient-dense, whole foods. Yet, it may curb your calorie intake excessively — and it can be difficult to maintain.

How the Biggest Loser diet works

Like many other weight loss diets, the Biggest Loser diet is a low calorie eating program. It also stresses regular exercise.

Its meal plans provide 1,200–1,500 calories per day and include 3 meals, plus 2–3 snacks from whole foods. The diet's guidebook claims that eating frequently helps keep you full, balances your hormone levels, and provides energy for regular exercise (1).

You're meant to plan and cook most meals on your own, carefully counting calories and weighing and measuring foods. You're further encouraged to keep a daily food log or journal.

Before starting the diet, it's best to calculate your individual calorie needs. Start by using an app or website to determine what you're currently eating.

For a safe 1–2 pounds (0.5–0.9 kg) of weight loss each week, subtract 500–1,000 calories from the number of daily calories you're currently eating and use that as your initial calorie goal.

Macronutrient composition

The diet stipulates that 45% of your daily calories come from carbs like vegetables, fruits, and whole grains, 30% from dairy and animal or plant protein, and 25% from healthy fats like nuts, seeds, and olive oil, as well as sugar-free or low sugar desserts.

The Biggest Loser 4-3-2-1 food pyramid provides a visual guide for the diet. It recommends:

- at least four daily servings of fruits and veggies (cooked and raw), plus a vegetable salad on most days

- three daily servings of protein from lean meats and fish, legumes, tofu and other soy foods, and low fat dairy products

- two daily servings of high fiber whole grains, such as brown rice, oats, or quinoa

- up to 200 daily calories from "extras," which include healthy fats, as well as treats and desserts

With its focus on nutrient-dense whole foods, especially fruits and vegetables, the Biggest Loser pyramid resembles the dietary recommendations from the U.S. Department of Agriculture (USDA).

SUMMARY

The Biggest Loser diet is based on the reality TV series of the same name. It's a reduced calorie eating plan that relies on whole, nutrient-dense foods meant to keep you feeling full throughout the day.

Does it aid weight loss?

Given that it slashes your calorie intake, the Biggest Loser diet should help you lose weight. You may experience even more benefits if you combine it with exercise.

However, you shouldn't expect the same results as the previous television show participants, who lost an average of 128 pounds (58 kg) over 30 weeks.

They did so by eating only 1,300 daily calories and engaging in over 3 hours of vigorous exercise each day with a trainer.

Various weight loss studies lasting 10–52 weeks indicate that low calorie diets result in an average weight loss of 22 pounds (9.9 kg) from diet alone. Those who add exercise experience a whopping 29 pounds (13 kg) of weight loss, on average.

The Biggest Loser diet is considered a moderate or balanced macronutrient diet, which means that it's not excessively high in protein, fat, or carbs. In fact, it adheres closely to the Acceptable Macronutrient Distribution

Range (AMDR) set by the Institute of Medicine.

Other popular types of weight loss diets include low carb or low fat diets.

In a yearlong study in 7,285 people comparing various diets, including the Biggest Loser diet, low fat and low carb eating patterns result in slightly more weight loss than moderate macronutrient diets.

However, all participants lost significant amounts of weight, regardless of their diet.

SUMMARY

If you follow the Biggest Loser diet's meal plans and exercise recommendations, you may stand to shed a significant amount of weight.

Other potential benefits

The Biggest Loser diet may have a few other benefits.

First, it may help you become a healthier eater because it incorporates whole, nutrient-dense foods and skips junk and fast food. It also stresses the importance of reading labels, measuring portion sizes, and keeping a food journal.

Using the Biggest Loser food pyramid to plan meals and snacks may likewise improve your diet quality. Researchers found this to be true for Americans who used the USDA's food pyramid to plan meals.

In fact, it may even reduce your cravings.

An analysis of 9 studies revealed that after 12 weeks, people who stuck to a low calorie diet had fewer cravings overall — and fewer specific hankerings for sweets, starches, and high fat foods.

SUMMARY

The Biggest Loser diet may curb your cravings for sweets and junk foods, as well as improve your diet quality.

Potential downsides

If you follow the Biggest Loser diet strictly, your daily calorie intake may be too low — especially if you're exercising intensely.

The authors recommend eating no fewer than 1,200 calories per day. However, for most men and many women, eating so few calories may leave you hungry and fatigued.

Furthermore, long term, severe calorie restriction may result in nutrient deficiencies that can trigger sensitivity to cold, the disruption of menstrual cycles, bone loss, and lower sex drive.

The diet is also heavily focused on reading food labels, counting calories, and eliminating high calorie foods. Occasional dining out is permitted, but it's essential to plan it into your daily calories.

Although these tips may all benefit weight loss, some people may find it time consuming, overly restrictive, and difficult to maintain — particularly in the long run.

Maintaining lost weight is a common challenge among weight loss programs, including the Biggest Loser.

In fact, the television show has received significant criticism not only for its drastic weight loss methods but also because contestants regained most of their weight upon followup.

Notably, it isn't unusual to regain half of the weight you lose in the first year after any diet program due in part to a slowdown in your metabolism. Also, many people slip back into old habits.

If you can maintain the diet long term, you'll have a better chance of losing weight.

However, research reveals that more people succeed at maintaining weight loss if they have some type of group or individual support, which the Biggest Loser diet doesn't provide.

SUMMARY

The Biggest Loser diet may be dangerously low in calories and overly strict or time consuming for some people. In addition, there's no one-on-one or group support available.

Foods to eat and avoid

This Biggest Loser diet emphasizes a variety of fresh, whole foods. Because few — if any — whole foods are banned and no foods are required, the plan is also flexible if you have dietary restrictions.

Fruits, non-starchy vegetables, and minimally processed whole grains will fill most of your plate. Starchy vegetables like sweet potatoes or squash are limited to just once or twice per week.

Protein choices include skinless poultry, leaner cuts of beef like sirloin or tenderloin, and seafood. Fattier fish, such as salmon and sardines, are encouraged for their omega-3 fats, but remember that they're higher in calories than lean fish.

Vegetarian protein options include all legumes, plus soy products like tofu and tempeh. Egg whites and low fat or fat-free dairy products, including milk, nonfat yogurt, and low fat cheese, are also recommended sources of protein.

You're meant to limit nuts, seeds, avocados, oils, and other high fat foods to only 100 calories per day.

The diet's only other limited foods are sweets, snack treats, and alcohol, which are restricted to 100 calories per day. In fact, you're encouraged to skip these extras and instead allocate the 100 calories to healthy food choices.

SUMMARY

The Biggest Loser diet provides a variety of low calorie, whole foods. You're able to eat from every food group but should closely monitor your intake of fats and desserts.

A sample menu for 1 day

Here is a 1,500 calorie menu for 1 day on the Biggest Loser diet.

Breakfast

- 1 whole grain toaster waffle with 1 tablespoon of fruit spread and 1 cup (123 grams) of raspberries

- 1 poached or boiled egg

- 1 cup (240 mL) of fat-free milk

Snack

- 2 ounces (57 grams) of smoked salmon

- 2 Wasa crackers (or a similar multigrain crispbread)

Lunch

- 1 small whole grain tortilla with 3 ounces (85 grams) of roast beef, 1 tablespoon of horseradish, lettuce, and 3 thin slices of avocado

- 1 cup (150 grams) of seedless grapes

- water or unsweetened iced tea

Snack

- 2 low fat mozzarella cheese sticks

- 1 large orange

Dinner

- 1 cup (240 mL) of fat-free lentil soup

- 1 serving of quinoa tabbouleh with tomato and cucumber

- 3/4 cup (128 grams) of sliced melon

- unsweetened tea

SUMMARY

A typical day's menu on the Biggest Loser diet includes three small, balanced meals and two snacks. You'll eat several servings of fruits and vegetables, plus lean proteins and some whole grains.

The bottom line

The Biggest Loser diet is a low calorie eating plan based on the reality television show of the same name.

It has been shown to aid weight loss by stressing meal planning, calorie counting, and portion control. Its meals are comprised of high fiber fruits, vegetables, and whole grains balanced with low fat proteins and small amounts of healthy fat.

Yet, it may dangerously restrict calories for some people and can be challenging to adhere to. What's more, there's no support during or after the program to help you maintain weight loss.

Still, if you're looking to eat healthy and shed weight at the same time, the Biggest Loser diet may be worth a shot.

Last February, "The Biggest Loser" host Bob Harper set out to his New York gym for a routine Sunday morning workout. It seemed like just another day in the fitness expert's life.

But midway through the workout, Harper suddenly found himself needing to stop. He laid down and rolled on to his back.

"I went into full cardiac arrest. I had a heart attack."

While Harper doesn't recall very much from that day, he was told that a doctor who happened to be in the gym was able to act quickly and perform CPR on him. The gym was equipped with an automated external defibrillator (AED), so the doctor used that to shock Harper's heart back into a regular beat until an ambulance arrived.

The chances of him surviving? A slim six percent.

He woke up two days later to the shocking news that he had nearly died. He credits his friend who had been working out with him, along with the gym coach, and doctor, for his survival.

Masked warning signs

Leading up to his heart attack, Harper says he hadn't experienced any of the common warning signs, such as chest pain, numbness, or headaches, though he did feel dizzy at times. "About six weeks prior to my heart attack, I actually fainted in the gym. So there were definitely signs that something was wrong, but I chose not to listen," he says.

Warren Wexelman, a cardiologist with the NYU Langone School of Medicine and Medical Center, says Harper probably missed other warning signs because of his peak physical condition. "The fact that Bob was in such amazing physical condition before his heart attack was probably the reason he didn't sense all the chest pain and shortness of breath that someone in not as great physical condition would have felt."

"Honestly, if Bob wasn't in the condition that Bob was in, he probably never would have survived."

So how did a 51-year-old man in such great condition have a heart attack in the first place?

A blocked artery, Wexelman explains, as well as the discovery that Harper carries a protein called lipoprotein(a), or Lp(a). This protein increases the risk of heart attack, stroke, and valve blockages. Harper most likely inherited it from his mother and maternal grandfather, who both died from heart attacks at 70 years old.

But while carrying Lp(a) certainly increases one's risk, many other factors go into increasing one's risk for a heart attack. "There's never just one risk factor for heart disease, it's multiple things," says Wexelman. "Family history, genetics you inherit, diabetes, high cholesterol, and high blood pressure all come together to make the picture of what we call heart disease, and makes the person — no matter if they are in the best shape, or worst shape — much more prone to having one of these events."

Facing and embracing recovery

 Share on Pinterest

Harper has made it his mission to address every underlying issue — from diet to routine.

Rather than approach each lifestyle change as a violation of his already healthful approach to fitness and wellness, he's choosing to embrace the changes he has to make in order to ensure a positive — and lasting — recovery.

"Why have guilt or shame about something that's completely out of your control like genetics?" asks Harper. "These are the cards that are dealt and you do the best you can to manage any condition that you have."

As well as attending cardiac rehab and slowly easing back into exercise, he's had to radically overhaul his diet. Before the heart attack, Harper was on a Paleo diet, which involves eating mostly high-protein, high-fat foods.

"What I realized after my heart attack was that my diet was lacking balance and that's why I came up with 'The Super Carb Diet' book," he recalls. "It's about being able to press the reset button and getting all the macronutrients back onto your plate — protein, fat, and carbs."

To help you take good care of your heart, we'll send you guidance on managing high blood pressure, cholesterol, nutrition, and more.

Helping other heart attack survivors

Though Harper tackled recovery — and the requisite changes to his lifestyle — with gusto, he admits that he was startled when he learned that having one heart attack puts you at increased risk for a repeat heart attack.

Indeed, according to the American Heart Association, 20 percent of heart attack survivors over age 45 experience a repeat heart attack within five years. And of the 790,000 heart attacks experienced in the United States each year, 210,000Trusted Source of those are repeat heart attacks.

Learning this reality only further emboldened Harper to take control of his body. "It was in that moment that I realized I was going to do everything and anything that my doctors told me," he says.

One of those doctor's suggestions was taking the medication Brilinta. Wexelman says the drug stops the arteries from reclogging and reduces chances of future heart attacks.

"We know that Brilinta is not a drug that anybody can take because it can cause bleeding," says Wexelman. "The reason that Bob is a good candidate for this drug is because he's such a good patient and people on these drugs really need to listen to their doctor who's caring for them."

While taking Brilinta, Harper decided to team up with the drug's manufacturer, AstraZeneca, to help launch an education and support campaign for heart attack survivors called Survivors Have Heart. The campaign is an essay competition that will see five heart attack survivors from all over the country attend an event in New York City at the end of

February to raise awareness for the warning signs of repeat heart attacks.

"I've met so many people since doing this and they all have a special and important story to tell. It's great to give them an outlet to tell their story," he says.

As part of the campaign, Harper coined six survivor basics to help other people who have experienced a heart attack face their fears and be proactive with their self-care — by focusing on mindfulness, as well as physical health and treatment.

"This is so personal and so real and organic to me, because I'm contacted by a lot of people who want tips on what to do after suffering a heart attack," he says. "Survivors Have Heart gives people a place and community to turn to for tips."

A renewed outlook

As far as where his story will go from here, Harper says he has no current plans to return to "The Biggest Loser" after 17 seasons. For now, helping others manage their heart health and avoid repeat heart attacks takes priority.

"I feel like my life is taking a turn," he says. "For now, with Survivors Have Heart, I have a whole other set of eyes that are on me looking for guidance and help, and that's exactly what I want to be able to do."

He also plans to advocate the importance of learning CPR and having AEDs available in public places where people congregate. "These things helped save my life — I want the same for others."

"I went through a major identity crisis this past year of having to discover new outlets in my life, and redefine who I thought I was for these past 51 years. It's been emotional, difficult, and challenging — but I'm seeing light at the end of the tunnel and feeling better than I have."

Get Screened for Stroke and Cardiovascular Disease Risk

Get screened for Stroke and Cardiovascular Disease Risk. Understand your risk through a simple, painless and non-invasive screening.

Get peace of mind or early detection

through Life Line Screening.